THE POSSIBLE DIET

Simple Strategies for Healthy Weight Loss

APRIL CAPIL

for Dr. G.
and Super Nova

Thank you for helping me believe -
in myself and my capacity
to change my story
and change my life.

That can't be possible.

I was staring at a number on a scale, and I could not believe it.

Only moments before, I had watched with increasing alarm as a nurse moved the 1-lb weight further... and further.... and then *even further* to my right, doing her best to balance it with the the three 50-lb weights that were already there. It still wasn't balancing, so after an almost apologetic pause, *she moved the 1-lb weight back and replaced it with a fourth 50-lb weight.*

Then she moved the 1-lb weight *another four spaces out.*

I weighed 204 lbs.

How was this possible?

Just six months before, I'd had a bilateral mastectomy with reconstruction - what I thought would be the most important thing I could do to reduce my chances of a breast cancer recurrence - but *despite a surgeon cutting off my muffin top to give me new boobs,* **I had somehow managed to put on six pounds.**

In that moment, I knew I had to change. I didn't know if I *could*, but I knew I had to **try**.

~

As a woman over 40 in America who's had a BMI over 30 for most of my life, I have been on a dozen diets. My weight over the last 30 years has slowly crept up 2 or 3 pounds a year, but I've always managed to hover somewhere between a size 12 and a size 16 (mostly a size 14) since I was in my 20s. I had the requisite suitcase full of clothes in my closet I hoped I would "someday fit in," but I had honestly given up on the idea of ever being "slim" or "athletic." I dreamed about it once in a while, of course - *maybe this plane will go down in the Pacific, and I'll survive, but be stranded on an island like Tom Hanks, which will force me to adopt a fish-and-coconut diet that will make me look like a South Beach Crossfit Goddess just in time to be rescued by a crew of Navy Seals!* - but I didn't *really* believe it was possible, so I had just... stopped trying. I'd accepted that I was always going to be a "*Big* Girl" and simply refused to let it stop me from accomplishing *BIG* goals - competing in an Olympic triathlon, running the New York Marathon, climbing Kilimanjaro, and walking the Camino Santiago. As far as I was concerned, I wasn't going to let society's unrealistic body image standards dictate what I could and couldn't do.

But there was that number, staring back at me.

At 204 pounds, with a BMI of 34, I wasn't just overweight. I was flirting with *Severely Obese* (which starts at a BMI of 35). And I knew - I **knew** that obesity was a contributor to not only cancer, but other life-threatening conditions, like metabolic syndrome and coronary heart disease. *Was this what I wanted?*

When I saw that number on the scale, all my rationalizations that a person can still be big and beautiful or fit and fat flew right out the window. I knew I was being dangerously naive about the consequences of carrying all that extra weight. What's worse, I was *lying* to myself, because in that moment, *I wasn't okay*. Not with my body, not with my choices. I was **scared**. I knew the road I was headed down, that was lined with positive body image slogans and stretchy jeans, could end in diabetes, or not being able to take the stairs without my lungs burning or my knees throbbing. Maybe not tomorrow, maybe not even this year, but someday, and probably within a decade or two.

I had to do something, even if it seemed **impossible**.

Two days later, I was in a doctor's office, filling out a form for a medically supervised weight loss program, despite firmly believing that **diets just wouldn't work for me**. What I *also* believed, though, was that thirty years of trying and failing to lose weight meant that I wasn't capable of doing it **without help**. If I was going to make a healthy, permanent change in my life, *I was going to need a professional*. I told myself that Michael Phelps didn't make it to the Olympics without a coach, and I wasn't going to be able to lose 50 pounds without one.

Dr. G. had the air of someone who had the same conversation a dozen times a day. Her tone was matter-of-fact as she talked about the things I'd need to do to lose the weight: reset my metabolism by stabilizing my blood sugar, get on a regular eating schedule, and cut back my calories by controlling my portions and eating more vegetables. Nothing she was telling me was new - I had heard it all before in one diet book after another - but this time, *I was paying attention*, because I honestly felt like my future was at stake if I didn't make a change.

She recommended a meal replacement diet, for a minimum of three months: two shakes a day, plus a low-carb meal and a vegetable snack. I would keep a food journal, meet with her once a week, and weigh in at every visit to monitor my body composition. She encouraged me to keep exercising if I enjoyed it, but warned me not rely on it for weight loss. Exercise, she explained, was good for flexibility and strength and endorphins, but it would be much easier to **cut** 500-800 calories a day from my diet than to ***burn*** 500-800 calories a day by working out. Dr. G. said if I followed her plan, I could expect to lose fifty pounds in somewhere between 6 and 12 months. This package was going to cost me $500 a month and it wasn't covered by my insurance. I swallowed hard. *This was going to be an expensive 50 pounds.*

I had never done anything like this before - a doctor-supervised program with meal replacement shakes? Would that even work for me? I thought of Oprah, losing all that weight from Optifast, then putting it all back on, and wondered if I would just be setting myself up for the same disappointment.

What sold me was a current of confidence, hovering underneath Dr. G's noncommittal tone. She was the picture of health, with an encouraging smile and kind eyes. There was no judgment, no drill sergeant hiding underneath her easygoing demeanor. I could tell she genuinely empathized with my struggles to accept my body, even as I desperately wished that I could change it. Here I was, coming to her trying to lose the weight I had been carrying for decades, and she was telling me with absolute certainty that it was not only *possible*, but it could take me less than a year to do it. She made it sound as simple as putting one foot in front of the other. Just like walking the Camino.

This is going to be harder than walking the Camino, though, I thought. *The Camino only took six weeks. This is going to take* **months**.

In addition to my own hangups about diets not working, bodies being beautiful at any size, and a simmering resentment that I was only changing my lifestyle to conform to societal norms, I knew I would be fighting an aging metabolism, a serious sweet tooth, and a lifetime of bad habits.

I considered my favorite Japanese proverb:

When is the best time to plant a tree?

25 years ago.

When is the next best time?

Today.

"Okay," I said. "I'm ready. Let's do it."

Looking back, I realized the biggest gift Dr. G. gave me wasn't a diet.

It was the idea that I could do something that I had never been able to do before.

Chapter One

THE CRACK

There's a crack that opens, somewhere in your brain, when it occurs to you that *something is possible*.

I've felt this crack open at least a dozen times in my life. I felt it when I saw Linda Francisco - a white haired roly-poly fairy of a woman - say "I've run three marathons!" and thought to myself, *"Well, if **she** can do it..."*

I felt it when my Ironman tenant Nicole said to me (a little too casually, looking back), "You could do a triathlon," and I found myself asking, *"Really? You think so?"*

I felt it when I read that Shirley MacLaine had walked the 500-mile Camino Santiago **at 60 years old**. *"Huh. She did it at 60?"* I mused. *"It must not be as hard as I thought..."*

This crack has always marked the beginning of undertakings that end up being my greatest adventures and accomplishments. It drives a wedge into some belief I have about what I can't - *what I couldn't possibly* - do, and then, weeks or months later, I am shaking my head in amazement at the top of a mountain, or on a paddle board in the middle of a lake, or taking a picture of a homemade almond croissant. I *thrive*, not just when I'm pushing the boundaries of what I think *I'm* capable of, but even moreso when I am giving other people evidence that makes them question what *they* think they're capable of. I love watching a stranger's face when I tell them about the time I kayaked a Class Three rapid on the Main Salmon or planned a chocolate tour of Paris with a dear friend, because I can almost hear the crack in *their* head, the moment they start to think, *"Maybe... I could do that..."*

The truth is, I kind of *like* being a crack dealer.

I like it because I know human beings are creatures of habit, and we *love* evidence. We seek it out, not just to support our belief systems, but to bolster the cases that we're trying to make - for why we can't do something, be something, or have something. We're very good at backing up these cases with **mountains** of supporting evidence... until *reasonable doubt* is introduced.

And *reasonable doubt* was the secret weapon Dr. G. had just given me, without even realizing it.

She had just cracked my brain.

Leaving her office, a million thoughts were swirling in my head as I built up evidence to support the idea that *this was possible. I mean, the woman had dozens of positive reviews on her website. Surely she knew what she was doing. They couldn't all be fake, could they? And two shakes a day? That would actually make meal planning a lot easier, right? I would only have to get one meal "right" a day. The other two meals would be no-brainers - shakes, almond milk, and vegetables. I could... I could do this, couldn't I? I mean, how hard could it be?*

Let me tell you: that first month was *hard*.

I'm a baker. I *love* baking. I can make fantastic things with sugar and flour and butter. And that first month, I wanted cake every day, and cookies every *other* day. My body *fought* me giving it less sugar, and sometimes, I lost the battle. But sometimes, I won. And eventually, I won **more** than I lost. Because the funny thing was, every time I had more than a hundred grams of carbs a day, I *didn't* lose weight, and every time I had less than a hundred grams carbs a day, I *did*. After a few weeks of taking two steps forward and one step back, it just started to seem **stupid** to derail all my hard work by indulging in a brownie sundae. Once I realized I could undo a week of clean eating with a plate of Fettuccine Alfredo and three glasses of wine, bingeing on pasta and Chianti started to look less and less appealing.

After a month of my brain trying to figure out what I could bake that would give me that "Nailed it!" Food Channel high but not totally take me back to square one, I just started baking *other* things. I hacked recipes and got creative, coming up with *healthier* recipes like spaghetti squash "pizza" and faux blueberry "danishes" so I could feel clever *and* stay on track. I got really good at making parmesan cheese veggie tacos and curries, and then every time I wanted something indulgent, I would add extra ice and a tablespoon of malted milk powder to my chocolate protein shake, or make a beautiful, colorful salad with homemade dressing. One time I even made a "pumpkin pie" protein shake when I was craving the Cheesecake Factory's signature Pumpkin Cheesecake.

When substitutes for my favorite treats didn't work, I used procrastination as my sugar-buster. I would put off making chocolate chip cookies until the weekend, and then forget about wanting them... or if I really wanted to make them, I'd have two, then bring the rest to work.

Having to hold myself accountable to Dr. G. with that meal log went a long way in curbing my unhealthiest habits. Sometimes what stopped me from eating a whole pan of snickerdoodles was not wanting to have to write "half a dozen cookies" in my food journal!

Dr. G. was always understanding and encouraging, and it wasn't until much later that I realized **she was modeling the way I should treat myself:** *with unconditional positive regard.* No judgment, no criticism, just an understanding and an awareness of what I was doing that was helping me reach my goals, and what I was doing that wasn't. She never let me beat myself up, and always encouraged me to just get right back on the horse. She helped me believe in myself, and my own agency, and reminded me on a weekly basis that underneath all my behavioral changes a *crack* was forming: a growing belief that it was *possible* for me to be someone who made different choices. That it was *possible* for me to **not** be a slave to my junk cravings. Just having confidence in my ability to break old habits and make new ones helped me keep my flywheel going, because once I **believed** there *was* a way, inevitably, **I found it.**

I had been in the habit of baking and eating sugary treats almost every week for decades, and it was not lost on me that this habit was one of the primary reasons I found myself where I was. Every week, Dr. G. reminded me that what I was trying to do was not just *lose weight.* My real goal - my long game - had to be **to disrupt the hormones and chemicals that had put my brain on autopilot for years.** I was going to do that rep by rep, by dismantling all the unhealthy habits that had been keeping my blood sugar on an insulin rollercoaster for most of my life. Once I did, I wouldn't turn to a box of brownie mix whenever I wanted to feel capable, or comforted, or celebrated. *These* were the real changes, Dr. G. assured me, that would enable me to not only lose weight, but to build a new, healthier autopilot to help me keep the weight off.

And you know what? **She was right.**

Thirty days after that horrible weigh-in, I had done something I thought was impossible: I *had lost ten pounds.*

I stared at the new number on the scale (*"Only three 50-lb weights!"* I squealed), and somewhere in my brain, *that crack deepened.*

This was possible.

~

Three months after I first started seeing Dr. G., my waist had shrunk so much that most of my pants didn't fit anymore, and the clothes I'd stuffed into the "when I lose weight" suitcase in my closet did.

And you know what? ***It felt good.***

It felt ***really*** good.

After a lifetime of wanting something that felt out of my reach, I began to feel like maybe I *hadn't* eaten myself into an inescapable corner. I thought maybe, with a little personal agency, it *was* possible to be the size I always felt I could be, deep down inside. That inane expression - *nothing tastes as good as thin feels* - rang in my head every time I drank one of my shakes, every time I passed up cake or ate salad instead of macaroni and cheese at a buffet. With every healthy choice I made, I knew I was reinforcing not just those neural networks that would support my new lifestyle, but the belief that *changing my body was possible*. In fact, it was **inevitable**, if I stayed the course.

I could do this.

Something as simple as changing what I ate gave me access to a Narnian wardrobe - a world I never even imagined I could live in, and a body I never thought I could have. As the weight fell off, I had no choice but to admit it was true. I had irrefutable proof.

Still, I wondered: could this all really be that... *simple*?

It *was*, even if it wasn't *easy*.

Chapter Two

SIMPLE, NOT EASY

Do the thing and you will have the power.

— RALPH WALDO EMERSON

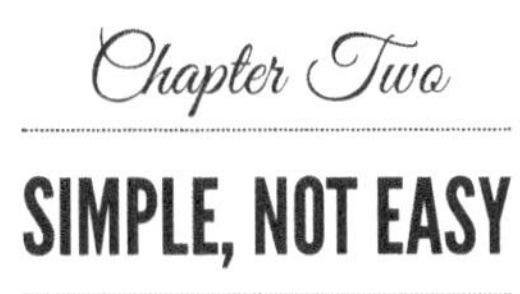

he problem I've always had with diets is **they are impossible.** Either the foods required are ridiculous, or expensive, or hard to make or hard to buy or hard to keep eating over and over and over. If a diet isn't prescribing impossible food *choices*, it's prescribing impossible eating *schedules* - forcing you to starve yourself for hours, or carry Tupperware containers everywhere, or avoid potlucks or restaurants. Most of them will demand a commitment to a life where you can never, ever eat at McDonalds or Panda Express or Cheesecake Factory *ever again.*

Ever? Really?

I could tolerate *impossible* for a week. Sometimes I could even tolerate it for a month (40 days during Lent if I *really* tried!). But then, after I lost a couple of pounds, or finally fit into my jeans again, or got injured working out, I'd fall off the wagon. I'd start sleeping in or Netflix bingeing instead of going to the gym. I'd get busy at work and find myself in a rut of eating rice and chili or macaroni and cheese, returning to the comfortable, easy foods I was familiar with. I'd indulge in dessert after I'd already had a pretty filling meal, or help myself to seconds because there was no Diet Angel on my shoulder wagging her finger at me to *"be good."* And after a few weeks of creeping back to my comfort zone one unhealthy choice at a time, I would start to feel out of control and helpless when it came to food, and resentful of a diet that was "impossible" to maintain.

~

I'll say it again: human beings are creatures of habit. This is because the lizard part of our brain equates safety and security with *what we know*, and "what we know" is everything from our past - all the habits and routines that have created millions of neural pathways that direct the flow of information like bullet trains. These neural pathways help us gravitate towards homeostasis - the most efficient state of being - because we conserve energy when we stay *where we are most comfortable.*

Change, on the other hand, is avoided, because it takes us away from homeostasis. When you eat less than you are used to eating, an alarm bell goes off in your brain, not because you *actually* need more food, but because you are diverging from your routine. Your brain is hard-wired to sound the alarm when you diverge from routine because somewhere in all that gray matter is a belief that *divergence will lead to discomfort.* That's all.

These biological signals are a neural safety net, existing solely to drive your behavior back to what is *familiar*, what is *known*, and what you are *in the habit of doing.*

In short, you are where you are because of things you have done, over and over, that have fired and wired all these neurons together, creating the "you" that behaves the same way in the same situations, time after time, *so you can feel safe.*

It's that simple.

You're not a bad person. You're not a stupid person. You're just a person who is in the habit of doing the same thing over and over.

The good news is, **you can break that habit.**

You would be *amazed* at how simple it is to break a habit - even a habit that feels like it has you in an iron grip. That habit exists because of a belief, and when you change your mind, you change your behavior. Break one little link in the chain reaction that keeps enforcing a habit and even something you have been doing for years will seem silly or inconvenient. When you adopt new beliefs, you will start to adopt new habits, and with repetition, they too will hold you in their grip, but it won't feel like a prison - it will feel *safe*, like a harness preventing you from falling off that wagon.

~

I joke that my superpower is that I'm an alchemist - I can turn lead into gold, lemons into lemonade. Through a lot of practice, I've gotten really good at managing adversity, changing my mind so I can change my expectations of myself.

The good news is, like Batman (and unlike Superman), I *learned* this talent, and *then* turned it into a superpower. I'm not any more gifted at transformation than any other human can reasonably expect to be, given enough practice and attention. What I've figured out is that once you can *believe something is possible*, making it a reality is just a matter of charting your course and laying down the bricks, or, as I've started to say lately, *doing the reps*. You may not do every rep, every time, every day, but if you do enough, eventually *you will get traction*. Once you get traction, you start to feel *agency*, and agency makes you feel *empowered*. Once you feel empowered, then all you want to do are reps, because agency is the most wonderful feeling in the universe. That's all **alchemy** is - <u>change over time, empowered by agency</u>. It looks like magic, but really, it's just transformation achieved through focus and persistence.

The hard part, of course, is the *believing*. Believing is the first step in transformation, and it takes time (and usually results) to convince a person that something is *really* possible. Humans often need overwhelming evidence to wrap our minds around a possibility, and even then, our minds will argue with equally convincing evidence to the contrary. If **not** believing something is possible makes our lives easier, we will deny it to preserve our homeostasis and justify avoiding discomfort.

For years, I believed that I couldn't change the size I was. I believed that surely, there was some complex process to losing weight that would never work *for me*. I believed that even if there was some quantum physics-level food-combining method or drug combination out there that *could* work for my body type, a person like *me* would never have access to it. So I resigned myself to a *belief*: that whatever could potentially unlock the mystery of "being thin" was probably only available to diet gurus or celebrities, and being thinner was just a physical impossibility for me. I blamed my DNA, my age, my metabolism, and my clearly genetic love of carbs, which was obviously why I had been a size 14 for twenty years. I knew - *knew* - that the "mystery" of why I couldn't lose weight couldn't possibly be as simple as **what I ate every day.** I knew this because I had been on a dozen diets where I changed what I ate, and <u>none</u> of them had worked! All these stories I told myself for years and years had convinced me that the solution to a lifetime of being fat *could just not be that simple.*

But it was.

It wasn't *easy* - it was a hundred smart decisions a day for weeks and months - but *it was simple.*

I replaced all my rice with cauliflower, broccoli, or greens.

I replaced all my pasta with zoodles or spaghetti squash.

I replaced all my crackers and bread with bell peppers and jicama, carrots or celery.

And when I did this, for a month, I lost ten pounds.

When I did it for three months, I lost 25 pounds.

It was that simple.

I started to believe that maybe, there wasn't anything "wrong" with me.

Maybe there wasn't anything "special" about me.

Maybe, the only thing standing between me and what I wanted... was *me*.

And because I wanted to believe this - because I wanted to start that chain reaction of *belief-reps-agency-empowerment*, I began collecting evidence to support that belief. I Googled "Weight Loss Transformations" and read stories about people -

hundreds of people - who had done the same thing: lost weight and transformed themselves. Picture after picture, diet after diet, I began to build support for an idea that I now had a mounting pile of evidence for: **I wasn't special.** *I was just like these people,* who had transformed their bodies and their lives simply by changing their behavior. *By doing the reps.*

They did something different, and got something different, just like me.

40 pounds lost later, I finally accepted that, like Dorothy, I had always had the power to change. There wasn't a secret trick, a magic drug, or a genetic advantage keeping me from being where I wanted to be.

I realized that, as Emerson put it, *having the power* was as simple as *doing the thing.* Again and again. Over and over.

It wasn't **easy**, but it *was* **simple.**

Chapter Three

FIVE HABITS

There were Five Habits I adopted during my diet that set me up for success. I found that when I maintained these habits, I lost weight, and when one of them started to fall by the wayside, my progress stalled until I picked up the habit again. They were:

- Pay Attention to Portions
- Don't Confuse Hunger With Something Else
- Eat More Fruits and Vegetables
- Move Every Day
- Practice Makes Perfect

I call these "Habits" because they are things I did every day, consistently, until they were as automatic as brushing my teeth. It **has** to be that automatic for you. In order to be a fit, healthy person, you have to *know* - the way you know the layout of the teeth in your mouth - what an appropriate portion of a food is, what the difference is between being hungry or being bored, and when you have gone too long without moving. Most importantly, you have to be able to see yourself as someone who is capable of getting where you want to be, just like I have, just like millions and millions of other people have, by doing the reps. Losing weight is not impossible. It's *possible*, with the right habits. It's **inevitable**, given the repetition of those habits over a period of time.

The good news is, these are simple habits and you can learn them. With practice, you can get better at them, until they are automatic and you don't even have to be conscious about them. Over the course of our time together, I told Dr. G. again and again, *"This process is rewiring my brain!"* because I could feel the change in my "autopilot" - the familiar, *habitual* response I've always had to a situation in the past. When my **beliefs** changed, my **behavior** changed, and when my **behavior** changed, my **brain** changed. It just got used to doing things differently. I actually *started to want different things*, to *crave* different things. And after years of always wanting something sweet after every meal (even breakfast!), I suddenly... didn't always want it. After years of feeling comforted by a stuffed stomach, that feeling started to make me feel sick and tired. Believe me when I tell you, the change you can make in your own thinking will be mind-blowing!

Just keep in mind, like Kelly LeBrock once said so famously, *"It won't happen overnight, but it will happen."* (#ThanksPantene)

HABIT 1: PAY ATTENTION TO PORTIONS

Do you know what a cup of something looks like? An ounce? A teaspoon?

Neither did I.

I *thought* I did, until I started measuring my food. What you think is a cup of pasta is probably a cup and a half, at least. What you think is a "tablespoon" is probably two, and the gigantic caloric difference between an ounce of cheese and an ounce of spinach might surprise you.

Fortunately, you don't have to worry about that just yet. It will be important later, when you're trying to lose those last ten pounds and you need to get militant about your portion control, but for now, all you need is your **hand.**

A portion of protein should be about the size of your **palm.**

A portion of fat should be about the size of your **thumb.**

A portion of carbohydrates should be about the size of your **closed fist.**

Portion control, when you're first starting out on this diet, is really that simple.

The hard part is realizing that you have probably been eating two or three (or four) portions of everything per meal, and now, you're going to have to cut back to *one* per meal.

The good news is, you can pretty much throw portion control out the window when it comes to *non*-starchy vegetables. Seriously, just *try* to eat five fists of broccoli or zucchini or spinach or kale or red cabbage or bell peppers. You'll be too stuffed to eat another bite long before you manage to consume too many calories of Romaine lettuce, trust me.

But for the *other* foods (like the Caesar dressing *on* that

Romaine lettuce), portion size *will* matter, and you're going to have to get used to controlling your portions if you want to lose weight. If cutting back to reasonable portion sizes sounds impossible for you - if you are someone who has been eating four palms of hamburgers in a sitting - *start with a small change.* Cut down to three palms in a sitting, then two, then one, until you get to a point where you can stop feeling hungry with just one palm-sized portion.

Notice how I said "stop feeling hungry" and not "feel full"? You're going to have to learn the difference between those too.

Which brings us to...

HABIT 2: DON'T CONFUSE HUNGER WITH SOMETHING ELSE

Another thing Dr. G. taught me is that if I listen to my body, it will tell me what it needs.

I know, I know: ***But what if my body is telling me it NEEDS Krispy Kremes?!***

Hold up, I'm getting there.

About a year ago, long before I got on this weight loss train, I took up meditating to combat stress I was dealing with at work. I couldn't just sit cross-legged for an hour in silence without my butt falling asleep, so I used "guided" mediations I found on YouTube instead. Many of them start with a "body scan" - a sort of walkthrough inventory of your body - to give you a chance to check in with yourself and prepare to relax. I got to really enjoy these guided meditations, and the more I did them, the more my brain started to feel "connected" to my body, like they were two friends dancing in the same space, rather than two armies battling for control.

In the past, I often confused hunger for other feelings - boredom, fear, anxiety, excitement, loneliness - and whenever I felt any of these things, I would look for something to eat. I wasn't *hungry*, but I was forcing my body to consume and digest food that it didn't need and wasn't ready for. My body, being accommodating, was like, *"Okay, she's eating, better process and store this for when we might need it later!"* And then, when I actually WAS hungry, I would starve myself out of some stupid desire to prove I had discipline. Those times, my body was like, *"HELLLOOOO?! I am not functioning at optimal levels! I need nourishment!!"* but I ignored it, denied it, and told it to shut up and stop being so needy already. It wasn't fair and it wasn't kind.

The more I strengthened the connection between my mind and my body, the more I understood the difference between *real* hunger - which is a signal that your gas tank is low and needs fuel - and all these other **fake** hunger signals. Fake hunger looks like this:

- You're **bored**, and eating gives you something to *do*.
- You're **stressed**, and eating gives you something to *distract you*.
- You're **scared**, and eating gives you something you can *control*.
- You're **lonely**, and eating gives you something to *comfort you*.

Eating is for one thing: *feeding your body and keeping it fueled and nourished.* **Hunger** is a signal that *you need to eat.* If you are already fueled and nourished, your body won't tell you it's hungry!

Also, you don't need to be *afraid* of hunger - hunger doesn't mean you are lame, or inept, or powerless, or alone. *It just means you need to eat something.* Plain and simple.

The next time you feel hungry, do a super-quick body scan to check in with yourself. Are you really **hungry**? Is that what this feeling is? Or are you just uncomfortable? If it's something other than actually being hungry, think about *what you really need*, not *what you want to eat*. Practice unwiring that neural pathway autopilot that's telling you, "Discomfort = Eating Something."

HABIT 3: EAT MORE FRUITS AND VEGETABLES

Dr. G. didn't worry so much if I had a chocolate chip cookie here or there, but she always expressed concern when my food journal showed a dropping off in my vegetable consumption. It was a sort of a canary in the coal mine - a signal that I was returning to my old unhealthy eating habits. She would always encourage me to have as many servings of vegetables as I could fit in a day, and I soon found myself adding spinach to an omelet or smoothie and having jicama or bell peppers as a snack. When you are trying to fit four or five servings of vegetables into your diet a day, there isn't much room for junk!

Berries also became my staples in summer, when they were readily available at my local farmer's market. I found myself looking forward to having raspberries or blackberries with cottage cheese or Greek yogurt, and even came up with a faux breakfast danish recipe to take advantage of all the fresh blueberries in season!

Fill your plate with lower-carb fruits instead of baked sweets and fresh vegetables instead of carb-heavy starches, and you won't have any room in your diet for junk. I always think of Christie Brinkley - still stunning even in her sixties - who credits her good health to *"going for as many colors as possible in a day!"*

HABIT 4: MOVE EVERY DAY

When the COVID-19 Shelter-In-Place order hit, that first week was rough. I was so sedentary that I was walking less than a thousand steps a day - I actually *put on* two pounds of fat, even though my weight didn't change! I realized that sitting all day was not going to be good - not for my joints, not for my ass, and certainly not for my metabolism - so I made a kind of "workout circuit" in my bedroom. I moved my mini trampoline behind my desk, then my Ab Roller between my trampoline and the door, then looped a resistance band over the door, and fixed a TRX-type band to my bathroom door. Every time I got up for a coffee or bathroom break, I'd do 50 High Knees on my trampoline, 10 Rollouts with my Ab Roller, 20 Reverse Good Mornings and 10 Low Rows off the TRX-type bands. This "obstacle course" made sure that I was able to stay active even when I was stuck indoors.

Of course, an in-home obstacle course/fitness circuit isn't possible for everyone. Even if all you can manage is a walk after dinner (or before breakfast!), fitting movement into your life will keep your body from atrophying, and open the door to a more active life. Move every day - your body will thank you for it.

HABIT 5: PRACTICE MAKES PERFECT

They saying goes, "How do you get to Carnegie Hall?"

Practice, Practice, Practice!

Practice makes perfect. Your brain is way more plastic than you think, and habits are built by reps - taking daily actions that fire and wire all those neurons together. The more reps you do, the stronger the connections in your brain get, and every time you reinforce a new pathway by repeating a new behavior, those old pathways start to atrophy. I like to say, you're always practicing something - are you practicing being a couch potato who eats junk food all day? If so, the more you practice, the better you're going to get at it! Think about what you want to be a pro at, and practice it relentlessly.

Never forget that every time you fire neurons together, they're going to wire together. If you've been *celebrating* with food or *comforting* yourself with food or *entertaining* yourself with food for 10, 20, 30 years, those neural pathways are **hard-wired**. It doesn't mean they're indestructible, but it does mean it's going to take a lot of reps to **un**wire them, and a strong alternative pathway. You're going to need to establish new behaviors for celebrating, comforting, and entertaining yourself *that have nothing to do with food.*

When you start building these new habits, **practice.** *Practice, practice, practice.* Every rep you get under your belt will strengthen those new neural connections and atrophy the old ones. After enough practice, those new behaviors will become automatic - you won't even have to think about it.

Chapter Four

HOW TO THINK

My greatest obstacle and greatest ally on this journey has not been my meal replacement shake, or my exercise routine, or even Dr. G.

It's been my **mindset.**

Getting your mind right is like putting your weight loss goals on autopilot. Your mind is the controller, the observer, the conductor and the director of your behavior, and how you respond to situations will determine if you are successful over time.

What always made diets impossible for me to stick to was *they felt like jail.* What I put my mouth has always represented my greatest, most enjoyable freedom. Maybe I couldn't *be* or do X, Y or Z, but I could *eat* whatever I wanted, whenever I wanted (never mind the *price* of all that indulgence!). For me, diets were always about *restriction* and *control* and *limiting* my freedom.

It's no wonder they never worked for me.

What changed my mind was the realization that **I wasn't**

free. I was slowly, with every pound I put on, *building a jail cell around me*. I was building my own prison, brick by brick, with each over-indulgence, each skipped workout, each depression-induced binge. I had been telling myself for years that the real damage to my happiness would be done by imposing unnecessary restrictions on my freedom, but I could not have been more wrong. The petulant parts of my personality were taking out loans on my future to finance fleeting comforts, not caring about that day twenty years from now when the bill for "treating myself" would come due. I was adding a bar to my cage with every unhealthy bite I took.

When I saw that number on the scale last year, it was like seeing a half-built wall of cinder blocks around me. I felt **trapped**: trapped in a body that was going to kill me. Trapped in a life where no one could see how beautiful I was inside because my outside didn't match it. Trapped in clothes that were too tight, and disappointed in myself every time I looked in a mirror. Suddenly, my brain saw my unhealthy behaviors for what they were: balms for wounds that had nothing to do with food. I was suddenly overwhelmed with **compassion** for my body, which was clearly struggling, despite years of mistreatment. This was the body that had fought cancer to give me a second chance at life, yet here I was, surrounding my organs with abdominal fat, letting my muscles atrophy, and justifying my behavior with arguments like, *"I deserve it!"*

"I deserve it?"

What a ridiculous idea.

I *deserved* health. *My body* deserved health. It deserved rest, and nourishment, and respect, and most of all, it deserved to be **loved**.

I decided right then and there that I would love my body like I love my 2-year old nephew: with empathy, respect, attention, and care. I would no longer restrict or abuse it, drown it in toxins to dull pain or stuff it into oblivion to blot out stress. That day with Dr. G., I embraced a simple commitment: to **pay attention**, and give my body the support it needed to be healthy for the rest of my life. Not to be healthy until I fit into a certain size; not to be healthy until I reached my goal weight, but *to be healthy for the rest of my life*. The alternative was... what? To be *unhealthy* for the rest of my life? **No way**, I decided. That was **not** going to be me.

And so, I went on a diet.

In the past, I associated a diet with prison, convincing myself that "freedom" was eating whatever and whenever I wanted, without any regard for my future. I assumed I had always been the same weight and would always be the same weight no matter what I ate, so what was the point?

The thing was, that number on the scale was telling a different story. My weight *wasn't* the same as it always had been - it was creeping up, slowly but surely. I was building a wall around my body with food, putting a layer between me and the world, and that layer was getting thicker. Soon it would smother me, committing me to a life sentence without the possibility of parole.

I'm convinced the reason why a diet worked this time was that for the first time, I saw the **possibility** of freedom from the prison I had built around me. I started to see myself as someone who could, through agency and empowerment, **change** my situation. Once I saw *the weight* as a prison and *my diet* as a tool I could use to escape it, I began to chip away at those walls, one pound at a time, like Andy Dufresne in *The Shawshank Redemption*. My desire for freedom - real freedom, lasting freedom - motivated me to make changes in my behavior. It motivated me to recalibrate my mind, to start seeing my diet as the path to a life where nothing could hold me back - not food, not fear, not self-consciousness or self-loathing. I stopped using food as a weapon, and started using it as a key - a key that would unlock my prison door.

~

*H*ere is a truth most humans know deep down in their heart of hearts: *no one can hurt you as much as **you can**.* There is no betrayal, no injury, no greater or more painful harm... than **self**-harm.

Consequently, there is no love more powerful, more nourishing, more restorative than self-*love*.

Your highest goal on this journey should be to **love yourself completely, all the time.** When you do this, you will not use food to punish or reward yourself. You will not need extra weight to protect or speak for yourself. Your body will be a testament to the kindness and empathy you have for yourself, because when you love yourself, you're good to yourself. It's that simple.

Self-love starts with self-care, and self-care starts with paying attention. I know - no one wants to open Pandora's Box. Weight is often the trauma we wear - that we put on, pound by agonizing pound - to protect a wound underneath. Losing weight may free you from a prison while simultaneously forcing you to face what put you in that prison - what you've been protecting yourself from. It can be scary.

By the time I had lost about 30 pounds, people wouldn't stop commenting on it. It was during the holidays and I was surrounded by friends I hadn't seen in months and buffets filled with food that was definitely not diet-friendly. Everywhere I turned, someone was either complimenting me while simultaneously caveating it with a *"Not that you didn't look great before!"* or encouraging me to "just take a break" from my diet and indulge. It was confusing and stressful, but the scariest part was, I felt like with every pound I lost, I was losing a little bit of myself. The feeling was weirdly reminiscent of when I was going through chemo - in both situations, I would look in the mirror and be startled to see someone different staring back. It would take me a minute to reconcile the "me" I *was* with the "me" I was *used* to seeing - the "me" I had been just a few months before.

What helped me get over this disorientation turned out to be the same thing that helped me stay focused on my goals: spending time every week visualizing where I wanted to be, through both meditating and journaling.

Some people can sit in a quiet space for an hour, contemplating their thoughts like a mountain yogi. That... is not me. Like losing weight, I found that having a coach to guide me through the process was really helpful. Whether you want music in the background or a soft voice walking you through a relaxation exercise, don't worry - YouTube has you covered! Here are a few of my favorite channels:

- The Mindful Movement - https://www.youtube.com/channel/UCu_mPlZbomAgNzfAUElRL7w
- Dexter and Alessandrina - https://www.youtube.com/channel/UCli47aB6PgEA7XibyS7GESA

- Rising Higher Meditation - https://www.youtube.com/channel/UCm1PrIQ1VmHHXAc8UlZTS9Q

If one-on-one classes are more your jam, Chris DiMeglio is another great teacher who offers online classes and webinars: http://www.chrisdimegliomeditation.com/

I also found the work of Dr. Joe Dispenza and Jose Silva to be helpful in creating a practice that helped me visualize the "me" I wanted to be, so I wouldn't constantly be thrown by how different I looked from the "old me." You can find a ton of guided meditations from Joe Dispenza and Jose Silva on YouTube, but... to be honest, most of them are bootlegs, so do an author a favor and look them up on Audible.com! :)

The key thing to remember is, your mind and body will seek alignment with whatever vision of yourself you hold in your head, so if you constantly see yourself as someone who is "always going to be thick" or someone who "couldn't possibly eat rabbit food," it's going to feel disorienting if every time you look in the mirror, your clothes are falling off you and you have kale between your teeth! Diverging from what you're used to can make you uncomfortable, and more likely to abandon this "new you" for familiar, comfortable "old you." To overcome this discomfort, you need to consciously, deliberately embrace the changes you're trying to make in your life, and get comfortable with the "new" you.

If meditation just doesn't work for you, you can try journaling instead. Whenever I found myself feeling lost or insecure, I would write a letter of encouragement, from "Future Me" to "Present Me." I would tell Present Me how proud I was of that I hung in there, how worth it it was in the end, because now, I could play tag with my nephew without stopping to catch my breath after five minutes, and find a gorgeous cocktail dress on short notice because I wasn't limited to the one size 14 that was left on the clearance rack. I would tell myself how thankful I was to make it to 20 years cancer-free, and be in better shape at 55 than I ever was at 25! I would write like I was writing to a best friend, to let her know I supported her, was pulling for her, and had faith she could do anything she set her mind to. It might seem silly, but never forget - *self-love is the best love!*

$\sim$

On this journey, anything different from what you are used to will feel uncomfortable at first. It might even feel scary. Remember, our minds are wired to associate divergence with danger. You have to believe that *it's possible for you to make different choices, and still be safe.* Hold a vision of you being free *and* healthy. Changing *and* thriving. Uncomfortable will become comfortable, with enough practice. You're learning something new, and eventually, it won't be new anymore. It will be *normal.*

What happens when you repeatedly and intentionally see yourself where you want to be is, your subconscious mind aligns your thoughts and actions to **figure out how to get there.** You'll start getting ideas that have never occurred to you before. You'll start trying things you've never tried before. You'll start rejecting thoughts and actions and behaviors that you know will derail you. And all of these changes? Eventually, they'll just be **who you are** and **how you live.**

That is the power of just believing *something is possible.*

Chapter Five

HOW TO EAT

Chandler Bing said it best, I think: *"A cookie is not a hug, Monica."*

For most of my life, food was my favorite kind of comfort. I *tried* to see it just as fuel, but the double curse of having a sweet tooth and being a good cook made it pretty challenging.

Plus, I. Love. Carbs. I mean, I *really* love them. Give me a bowl of hot buttered noodles with a little parsley, garlic and chili? Oh my God, I'm in Heaven. Pound cake? Yes, please. And bread? Don't even get me started on warm, crusty, buttered sourdough. I'm a Californian! That stuff is my kryptonite.

The first thing I learned from Dr. G. was that simple, starchy carbs are not my friend. If I wanted to not be at risk for everything that comes with obesity, simple carbs were going to have to be *very special treats*, consumed on *rare occasions*. And she meant **all** of them: sugar, sweets, bread, pasta, rice, tortillas, crackers, pretzels.

Pretty much everything I enjoyed eating on a regular basis.

But, that's how I got into this mess, right? I had literally built a gingerbread jailhouse around me, covered in frosting and candy. I had no one to blame but myself.

Did I mention I'm half Filipino? I grew up eating white rice *every single day*. Except when we had spaghetti. True story: the first time I ate dinner at a white friend's house and saw a plate of Wonder Bread stacked on the table, I said, *"Where's the rice?"* They looked at me like I was nuts. My friend shrugged and said, "We only eat rice with Chinese food?"

Anyway, back to carbs.

I had been using carbs for comfort for almost 40 years, and Dr. G. was telling me they no longer belonged in my diet - at least not in the amounts I was allowing them to be. She said if I wanted to not only lose weight, but keep it off and live a long, healthy life, I had to think of ways to replace all the simple carbs I was *used* to eating with a lower-carb fruit or vegetable, and save the real thing for special occasions.

Again: simple, but not easy.

So, I started one carbohydrate at a time.

First, I stopped eating bread, rice, or pasta every day. When I wanted bread, I would have a baked or oven-fried sweet potato. It was starchy and comforting, but had a lower glycemic index, and wouldn't spike my blood sugar if I ate it with some grilled steak, light butter, green onions, and nonfat Greek yogurt. It wasn't a trip to Outback Steakhouse, but it was close, and way healthier.

When the holidays came, I started bringing sliced up bell peppers to parties, so I could enjoy the spinach artichoke and buffalo chicken dips. Usually by the time you eat two bell peppers and a half a cup of dip, you don't have much room for warm sourdough bread!

I tried spaghetti squash, which I've apparently been over-cooking most of my life. Once I got it right, it became my new favorite comfort food. Hot spaghetti squash with a little pesto? So good! And even better without the guilt or carb coma that usually follow a giant bowl of pasta.

The Big Boss of my battle was, of course, baked goods. I mean, I make a fantastic chocolate chip cookie, and I tried every-thing - protein flour, low-carb, sugar substitutes, all of it - but nothing was as good as the real thing. So sometimes, I had the real thing. Sometimes, I had sugar-free chocolate chips and 20 almonds instead (although, Dr. G. once shook her head at my food log and said, *"You shouldn't even bring nuts in the house!"* because it's so easy to eat 500 calories' worth if you're not paying attention). Sometimes, I just had a bowl of raspberries and cottage cheese.

When you *believe it's possible* to navigate your days without being controlled by when and where you are going to eat your next chocolate chip cookie, your brain figures out *how to do just that*. Bingeing on sweets and keeping your blood sugar stable are mutually exclusive. The more time you spend off that insulin rollercoaster, the less time you want to spend on it. I didn't "kick" sugar, and I didn't cut it out of my life. I just moved it to a corner where it doesn't get in the way of my health.

Protein and Fat, I learned, **are** my friends. My challenge with Protein has always been eating enough of it, and getting used to having it at every meal. With Fat, I was so phobic of its calorie density (120 calories in a tablespoon, typically) that I went through a phase on my diet where I actually cut back on it, but found myself starving and craving carbs as a result. As soon as I put the fat back in my diet, I felt more satiated and stopped dreaming about layer cake. So make sure you get enough protein, and don't be afraid of fat.

Lastly, get ready to meet the new loves of your life: Fruits and Vegetables. You are probably going to have to triple your intake of vegetables for this diet. Don't be scared - it'll be unfamiliar waters at first, but once you get the hang of it, it'll seem weird to *not* have them with a meal. Start by swapping your muffin or danish with a low-carb fruit (always with a Protein or a Fat) at breakfast. Have a side of veggies at lunch and dinner, then two sides, then three, until veggies are at least half your plate. You won't regret it! Make these choices again and again and they will become automatic. Better yet, remove the choice in the first place - fill your cart with produce at the grocery store or your local farmer's market, so it's the first thing you reach for at home. These days, I have five, six, seven kinds of fruits and vegetables in my fridge at all times, and even more in my freezer! In a pinch, I know I can always steam some frozen broccoli and pan-fry a Trader Joe's pre-formed burger patty (which don't just come in beef, by the way - TJ's sells turkey, salmon, tuna, bison, and even shrimp burgers!). Being prepared with plenty of fruits and veggies available keeps me from staring at the box of Velveeta Macaroni and Cheese (thankfully collecting dust) in my cupboard.

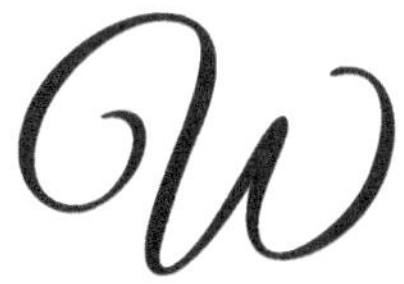

hen it comes to food, half the battle is just *paying attention*. You can't have three helpings of Osso

Buco and eight glasses of wine if you want to lose weight. You know this. You may be in **denial** about this, but you *must* know this. You might be able to get away with four glasses of wine once a year on your birthday, but you can't have four every weekend, or you're going to be drinking yourself into an early grave.

And let me just ask: *Is that what you want?* It can't be, or you wouldn't be reading this book, right?

Paying attention to what you're putting in your mouth is the first food choice that's going to make everything else possible. Read labels, log your meals, and pull away the veil that you've allowed to exist between you and the food you're eating. It's going to be scary, and maybe even heartbreaking (like the day I realized that my favorite bowl of ramen has 62 grams of carbs in a serving), but being aware of **how the choices you have made led you to where you are** is going to empower you to make *different* choices.

Making *different* choices, as it turns out, is the only thing that can give you *different* results.

HOW TO MOVE

A person can do anything for 30 seconds.

— LOU KRISTOPHER, BOOT CAMP COACH

D r. G. was right: it is way easier to cut 500-800 calories out of your diet every day than it is to *burn* 500-800 calories a day through exercise.

Don't believe me?

Average calories burned per hour of exercise (for a 200-lb person):

- **Walking** 2 mph: 255 calories per hour
- **Yoga**: 228 calories per hour
- **Canoeing**: 319 calories per hour
- **Riding a Bike**: 364 calories per hour
- **Skiing** or **Golfing**: 391 calories per hour (IF you carry your clubs)

- **Aerobics** or an **Elliptical**: 455 calories per hour
- **Swimming**: 528 calories per hour
- **Running** 5 mph: 755 calories per hour

I don't know about you, but I can't run an hour a day, *every single day*, for *months*. If I tried to, you can bet I wouldn't also be able to keep my calorie consumption reasonable.

Dr. G. reassured me that exercise wasn't *necessary* for me to lose weight, but it would definitely be **good** for me while I was trying - it could release endorphins, keep me limber, improve my heart health and give me more energy. In addition, because I also incorporated strength training into my routine, I would be staving off osteoporosis and improving my balance. In her eyes, exercise was a win-win, as long as I didn't use it to justify overeating on my "workout days."

How many days did I workout every week while I was trying to lose weight? *Three.*

That's it. Two one-hour gym sessions and one day where I walked my nephew in a stroller, or hiked with a friend, or took a yoga class.

I know it sounds unbelievable, but I didn't need to spend hours doing Crossfit or Zumba or playing water polo to lose weight. You can if you like, but don't depend on it as a substitute for restricting your calories or a justification for eating more.

My gym workout was pretty simple: I warmed up on a rowing machine for 1000 meters, then did pull-ups on an assist machine interspersed with squats, followed that with a HIIT Tabata session on a spin bike for 15 minutes, then cooled down for 20 minutes walking on a treadmill. The whole routine took just under an hour.

When the COVID-19 Shelter In Place order hit, I was still about 20 pounds away from my goal weight, so after the gyms closed and I was forced to work from home, I would do 50 "high knees" on my trampoline every couple of hours, take a walk during lunch, and do bodyweight exercises with a resistance band every other day to stay active. I even dusted off my Ab Roller and invested in a set of imitation "TRX"-type bands, courtesy of Amazon.

The best gift I got from losing weight came when I was 40 pounds down: I was able to take up running again.

Okay, I can hear your collective groan, but here's what happened: it was a beautiful day - one of those California Saturdays that just look like a postcard - and I went outside and thought, *"Man, this would be a great day for a run..."*

Then, I immediately thought, *"It's too bad I can't run anymore."*

You see, six years ago, I threw my back out so bad I could barely walk. It felt as if I had a shard of metal stuck in between my pelvic bone and my spine, right behind my hip. The pain was was *excruciating*. Eventually, a doctor told me I'd herniated a disc, and my options were back surgery (not recommended for someone who'd just turned 40) or long-term pain management with opiates (not recommended for anyone, really). I didn't like either option, so he suggested I give up running, take up yoga, and avoid sitting or standing for more than a few hours at a time. With time and rest, he said, it was possible my body could recover on its own.

It took me years to work up to it (and a lot of massage therapy), but I finally got my back strong enough to do a squat - no minor feat. And that day, when the sun was shining and a breeze was blowing, I laced up my sneakers and went for a tentative jog, trusting my back could handle it if I took it easy.

Wouldn't you know it - running is actually *enjoyable* when you're not carrying the equivalent of an Arrowhead water cooler bottle on your back!

Being able to do something I thought I'd never be able to do again has truly been the best part of losing weight - better than fitting into my clothes, or being more comfortable in an airplane seat, or even knowing the next time I draw my blood for a physical I won't be embarrassed by the numbers and full of excuses for my doctor.

I'll go into more details on my workout plan in the next chapter, but for now, just think of what you can do to *get moving*, three times a week. You don't even have to go to the gym - there are literally dozens of free bodyweight workouts on YouTube! If pushups scare you, can you walk? Try walking a mile (20 minutes), or even half mile (10 minutes). When I was going through chemotherapy, sometimes it would take me almost half an hour to walk a mile, and sometimes, that mile was all I could manage! But one day in the gym, I read an article about the New York Marathon, and put it on my bucket list. I worked up to it, one mile at a time, and two years later, I crossed the finish line. I still get choked up when I think about where I started from, and how good it felt to make a dream come true.

What first step are you willing to take today, on your journey of a thousand miles?

Chapter Seven

MY FOOD & FITNESS PLAN

In the age of information, ignorance is a choice.

— JOE DISPENZA

Everyone has a different amount of weight to lose. This diet is just a description of how I lost 55 pounds in ten months by changing my eating and committing to moving. You should **always** check with a doctor before starting any weight loss or exercise program, because there may be things about your particular health situation that aren't compatible with this food and fitness plan. A doctor can help you set realistic weight loss goals, and monitor your progress to ensure you're losing weight safely and at a reasonable pace.

Transparency was my Achilles' heel when I first started seeing Dr. G. In the beginning, I wrote down what I ate and the portions I was eating, but I didn't really know how on- or off-track I was until I started using a food-tracking app. I used

MyNetDiary, but many people like My Fitness Pal or Noom, or even Weight Watchers!

A food-tracking app is the best way to track your calories, and you're going to need to track your calories to lose weight.

There's no getting around this. "Calories in - Calories out" is a big part of what will help you reach your weight loss goal. It does you no good to follow the guidelines I've laid out in this book but be way over your allotted calories because you're not aware of how many you're actually eating. Use whichever app you like best, but it's worth it to get one that has a large database of foods and allows you to enter your current weight and a weekly weight loss goal. Start with trying to lose 1-2 pounds a week and adjust this if it feels too restrictive - remember, slow and steady sets you up for success! Don't forget to update your weight weekly and enable the app to adjust your calories accordingly. A good app will automatically calculate the number of calories you need to eat (including your macros) to lose the weight you want to lose, at the pace you want to lose it. A *really* good app will warn you when you set unrealistic goals, like a calorie budget of 700 (or 7,000) a day.

On my diet, I used MRPs (Meal Replacement Products) to keep my calories down and macros perfect. I used Wio's "PRO-22, Phase 1-3" shakes, which are typically only purchasable through a doctor, but here is the nutritional profile, if you choose to use a similar MRP shake on your plan: https://www.e-medtek.com/wio-mrp-meal-replacement-protocol-shake-vanilla-pro-22-phase-1-3-21-serving-bag *You do not have to use a Meal Replacement Product if you don't want to.* I had equally positive results losing weight on days when I replaced my MRPs with real meals; using MRP shakes just made it easier for me to get in a perfectly calibrated meal with very little time and effort. Even now, I still have a shake almost every day to make sure I'm getting enough protein, fiber, and nutrients in my body. It's a lifesaver when I'm traveling or don't have time to cook!

Regardless of how you're meal planning, remember the Five Habits that will make your weight loss possible - monitor your portion size using your hand as a guideline (a thumb's worth of Fat, a palm's worth of Protein, a fist's worth of Fruit or Starchy Veggies, or two fists' worth of Non-Starchy Veggies). **Think** before you help yourself to seconds - are you really still hungry, or are you just not used to eating a smaller portion size yet? You can expect to be hungry sometimes - you are training your body to eat less, and it's going to take some time for your brain and stomach to get used to it. But don't be afraid of being hungry, and don't confuse feeling hungry for feeling something else, like boredom, anxiety, or loneliness. *If you're not hungry enough to eat a bowl of steamed broccoli, you're probably not really hungry!*

MY FOOD PLAN

BREAKFAST

General Rules: If you have tea or coffee, or aren't that hungry, have one serving each of of a low-carb Fruit and Protein. If you're still hungry, have 16 oz. of water and wait 20 minutes before having seconds. If you find yourself constipated, you can add 1 Tbsp organic apple cider (with the "mother") to a glass of water or sugar-free flavored sparkling water. Alternatively, I've found that a sugar-free powdered magnesium supplement can also help (usually 300 mg a day, also mixed into water).

Fat: 1-2 cups tea or coffee with cream/half-and-half and/or sugar substitute (no real sugar - I use erythritol, allulose, monkfruit, or stevia)

Protein/Fat: eggs/egg whites, non-fat or low-fat Greek yogurt, non-fat or low-fat cottage cheese, nuts or nut butters or cheese (stick to no more than 1 Tbsp worth - nuts are very high-calorie!)

Carb: any kind of berries, stone fruits (apricots, plums, nectarines, peaches), apples, pears, or citrus (whole fruits, not juice)

Alternate Fats/Veggies: if you're not having coffee with cream, you can have a little butter or olive oil or cheese with your egg, or scramble in some leafy greens or other veggies.

LUNCH AND DINNER

General Rules: The easiest lunch for me is steamed or roasted veggies with a chicken-based curry, or a salad with grilled fish or chicken, but as long as you have one serving of Protein and 1-2 servings of leafy greens or vegetables (limit Starchy Veggies to 1 serving) with a little fat, you'll be satiated.

Greens: pre-mixed salad or broccoli slaw, spinach, kale, chard, collards, bok choi, red/green lettuce or cabbage

Steamed, Baked/Roasted or Stir-Fried Veggies: broccoli, cauliflower/cauliflower rice, zucchini, summer squash, onions, peppers, mushrooms, carrots

Starchy Veggies: sweet potatoes, beets

Proteins: eggs/egg whites, chicken, turkey, grass-fed beef or bison/buffalo, seafood (fresh or canned fish, shrimp, crab)

Fats: Primal Palate or Bolthouse salad dressings, olive oil or grass-fed butter, avocado or nuts/nut butters (watch those portions!), cheese in small (< 1 oz.) amounts

<u>SNACKS</u>

General Rules: Have a snack if you need it. If you don't, feel free to skip it. Keep your snacks under 200-300 calories - remember, it's a Snack, not a Meal. You can either follow the same guidelines above for Breakfast, Lunch and Dinner, and just cut the portion size in half, or you can eat something completely different. I like Larissa's Jerkies, Whisps Cheese snacks, jicama with baba ganoush, red bell peppers with seasoned Greek yogurt, or even a chicken drumstick in a pinch! Fresh fruits are fine but stay away from dried fruits - **carbs are super-concentrated in dried fruits**, and while they have a tad more fiber than Girl Scout Cookies, *many have just as much sugar.* One cup of sweetened dried cranberries, for example, has practically the same nutritional profile as *a bag and a half of Skittles!*

MY FITNESS PLAN

As I mentioned in the previous chapter, I really only "worked out" twice a week. I would leave room in my schedule for a third day of "moving" - either going for a walk, taking a yoga class or hiking, but I wasn't killing myself in the gym - just getting my heart rate up and trying to build muscle and improve my balance. If you really want to get stronger and fitter with the support of a professional, seek out a personal trainer! I'm not a gym rat and definitely not an expert; I'm just sharing what I did, that worked for me.

For the exercises below, feel free to break it up into however many sets you need to get through everything, e.g., 30 reps can be broken up into 6 sets of 5 or 3 sets of 10 or 2 sets of 15. Start with the low number and work up to the high one. When you get to the point where you're no longer feeling challenged, up your weight or resistance level and then start back at the lowest number of reps again. Alternatively, if even the lowest number of reps is too challenging for you, feel free to cut the complete routine in half and work your way up to it slowly over time.

MY GYM WORKOUT

Warm-Up: 1000 meters on a rowing machine (usually takes 5-6 mins)

Strength Training: Three sets of 8-12 pull-ups on a pull-up assist machine (if your gym doesn't have one of these, substitute push-ups or incline pull-ups on a Smith machine) interspersed with three sets of 15-25 squats (if you have lower back or knee issues, you can skip completely, or try lunges, or use a resistance band to take the weight off your knees and back until you can do them unassisted)

Cardio: 15 minute 20/10 "Tabata" session on a spin bike. Tabata is a form of High Intensity Interval Training (HIIT) where you "work" at an intense pace for 20 seconds, then "rest" at a less intense pace for 10 seconds. I always start my Tabata with a 90-second warm-up pedaling at a reasonable pace, then pedal 20 seconds at a faster pace, rest for 10 seconds, then do another 20 seconds fast, 10 seconds rest, and so forth, until I've done 24 rounds (20 seconds + 10 seconds = one 30 second "round" x 24 = 12 minutes total HIIT). I then cool down on the bike for another 90 seconds.

Cool Down: 10-20 minutes walking on a treadmill at a 2-4 mph pace.

MY AT-HOME WORKOUT

When the COVID-19 Shelter In Place lockdown hit, I had to get creative, so my workouts got a little messy for a while. At first, I took free classes on Amazon Prime, but I have a pretty tiny living room, which made all those grapevines challenging! After a healthy bit of Googling "At-Home Workouts" and "Bodyweight Exercises," and trying a few different ones, I finally managed to put together a home routine that I was comfortable doing a couple of times a week. I started with just two circuits of 10 reps each and am working my way up to 3 circuits of 20 reps each! Eventually, I got in the habit of also running or walking 30-40 minutes once or twice a week when the weather was nice.

My At-Home Strength Training Routine (2x/week on non-Cardio Days):

Circuit 1:

Warm up with 5 minutes of dancing (I'm totally serious - I just put on some Beyoncé or J-Lo or Justin Bieber or Taylor Swift and shake it out!) or 30-50 high knees with air punches (you could probably also do jumping jacks or mountain climbers)

1. 10-20 Walking Lunges
2. 10-20 Jump Squats
3. 10-20 Push ups (use knees if necessary)

4. 10-20 Side Planks (hold 10-20 secs), or Hip Thrusts or Glute Bridges

Repeat Circuit #1 2-3 times, resting 60 seconds between each round, then start Circuit #2

Circuit 2:

1. 10-20 TRX-type Single Leg Squats (each leg)

2. 10-20 TRX-type Rows

3. 10-20 Lateral Side Lunges (each leg)

4. 10-20 Step-Ups onto a bench

5. 10-20 Straight-Leg Sit Ups

Repeat Circuit #2 2-3 times, resting 60 seconds between each round, then Cool Down

Cool down with a Stretch Circuit (Quad Stretch, Hamstring Stretch, Hip Flexor Stretch, Deltoid Stretch, Tricep Stretch, Glute Stretch)

If the above routine down't work for you, that's okay! Honestly, *the Internet has already figured this out.* Check out any of the amazing stay-at-home-moms, fitness icons, and personal trainers on <u>Shape</u> or <u>Oxygen Magazine</u>'s websites (my favorites are Jamie Eason and Erin Stern), who gladly share their At-Home Bodyweight Workouts for readers who can't get to a gym or buy expensive equipment:

- https://www.oxygenmag.com/workouts/bodyweight-workouts
- https://www.shape.com/fitness/workouts/bodyweight-training

Chapter Eight

SNAGS AND PLATEAUS

It's inevitable. You are seeing results, staying on track, and then... everything grinds to a halt.

When you find yourself stalling, you might need to get a little technical, especially if you are hitting the dreaded "plateau." When I had lost 35 pounds and was trying to lose my last 15, I had to get really serious about tracking calories and macros to move that needle. *Any* time I had pasta or a cookie or a glass of wine, the number on the scale just wouldn't budge. It took me four months to lose those last 15, because I could no longer get away with a piece of bread here or a cup of rice there anymore. I had to stay on top of my portion control and do strength training or cardio three times a week, taking my vitamins every day instead of just when I remembered to.

If your progress stalls, the first thing you should double-check is whether you are being accurate about your macros and calories. Was that *really* a **half** a cup of rice? Or... was it more like a **whole** cup? Did you *really* only eat 20 tortilla chips, or did you just stop counting at 12 and ballpark it when the bowl was empty? This stuff matters when the margin of error can mean the difference between losing half a pound a week and putting on a pound.

If you're trying everything and the scale still won't budge, try restricting the hours you eat. I got in a bad habit during Shelter-In-Place of grazing all day, spacing out my calories over 17 or 18 hours, from the moment I woke up to right before I went to bed. I was eating the same amount of food, but my digestive system barely had any time to rest before I was putting it back to work again. To break my grazing habit and give my system a solid recovery period, I restricted my "feeding window" by eating my three meals and a snack between around 8:00 a.m. or 9:00 a.m. to about 6:00 p.m. or 7:00 p.m., depending on when I was planning on having dinner. This gave my body a 14-hour window where it could rest and repair itself without having to process any food. After a couple of weeks, the scale started to budge and I began losing steadily again.

Another thing I did was have a tablespoon of apple cider vinegar in 10 ounces of flavored sparkling water in the morning when I woke up, and again at night right after dinner. This served a two purposes. First, it gave me something to put in my stomach during that hour between waking up and eating breakfast, so I wasn't starving at the tail end of my "fasting window." Second, it increased the amount of water I was drinking every day by about 50%. The funny part was, it actually became kind of like my healthier substitute for a cocktail! I got weirdly into it, trying all kinds of flavors to find a mix I really liked (ginger and lime was the winner - it reminded me of a Moscow Mule).

$\mathcal{E}$ven if you're being militant about your macros, avoiding late-night snacks, and staying away from alcohol, the most powerful tool you have for overcoming snags and plateaus is going to be.... you guessed it: **your mindset.** Staying motivated when you're digging to China isn't easy - it's monotonous, and even when you can recognize how far you've come, sometimes it's discouraging to think of how much further you still have to go. To maintain the enthusiasm and commitment you'll need for the long haul, you're going to need a nice balance of inspiration and celebration.

To inspire yourself, find stories like yours, either through a support group of like-minded people struggling with the same challenges, or online stories of people who have succeeded after overcoming similar struggles. This works for anything in life - you can always find inspiration in a shared journey. Here are a few resources that inspired me:

- https://www.boredpanda.com/before-after-weight-loss-transformation
- https://www.oxygenmag.com/fat-loss/success-stories
- https://www.menshealth.com/transformations/

Stories like these gave me confidence, because they reminded me I wasn't doing something impossible - I was doing something that many, many people have done - people who often had bigger challenges and harder obstacles!

To celebrate yourself, **don't use food.** I know you want to! I wanted cake and ice cream the day I hit my goal weight - not because I was actually craving it, but because.... well, what else would you celebrate with?! Knowing it would immediately put me over my goal weight, I passed up the cake and instead went for a walk in the sun.

I paid attention to everything on that walk - the air, the heat, but especially my shadow on the ground, which I had worked so hard, for so long, to change. I marveled that **that was me**, reflected on the sidewalk. That was **my body**, that I had remade into a healthier, freer version of itself - the body that was going to carry me into a ripe old age without metabolic syndrome or coronary heart disease. I walked with the sun shining on my face, feeling how comfortable my clothes were and how strong my back felt. Like Walt Whitman, *I celebrated myself and sang myself*. I made a sonnet of that day, and set myself to music. My heart was open and happy, filled with gratitude for all the steps I took, and all the reps I did, to get myself there.

Chapter Nine

THE GREAT EIGHT

There have been a lot of "life strategies" I've learned in the last decade - most of which I've documented in my previous books, *Recipe For Lemonade*, *Life After Lemonade*, and *New Tricks*, but this last year I feel like I kept coming back to something new - something I've started referring to as my "Great Eight."

My Great Eight came out of a conversation I had with Dr. G. about the importance of routine, and the simplicity of a life that is architected for success. Success doesn't come from getting access to rich or powerful people or places, from having lots of fame or money. **Success comes from reps.** And reps are just **habits** - rinsing and repeating, staying on track.

If you've ever read *The Power of Habit*, you know that habits that are easily triggered and easily repeated are easy to maintain. What Dr. G. kept pointing out (man, she's good!) is that one easy way to reinforce a habit is to just write it down and post it in a place you can see it every day. It becomes a visual trigger to check in and make sure you are doing something you know will keep you on track. She asked me to write down the most powerful habits I've adopted that keep me on track and never fail to improve my quality of life, and then post them in a place where I can see them every day. I started with four, which turned into six, and finally, settled on eight. My **Great Eight** are the habits that I can rely on to keep me healthy, happy, and set up for success.

When something is off, when I don't feel good, when I'm cranky or depressed or feel awful physically, I come back to these eight things FIRST. Without fail, when I start doing them all again on a regular basis, I feel better.

MY GREAT EIGHT

#1: Sleep. Get 7-8 hours of sleep every night. This is my #1 habit. Without it, everything else falls apart. ***You have to find a way to give your body the time it needs to rest and repair itself.*** Running at full speed with no downtime is a recipe for disaster, and chronic sleep deprivation can really hurt you - more than you may realize. Studies have shown that not getting enough sleep increases your risk factors for every major health issue, so do yourself a favor and make this your #1 priority.

#2: Exercise. Move at least 30 minutes every day. Sweat if you're up to it. Exercise is pretty much the only thing most scientists will agree on is a "magic pill" for making everything in your life better, even if they can never agree on the type or frequency. Just walking 30 minutes a day provides enormous health benefits compared to laying on the couch all day! If you want to get your heart rate up and do some strength training, try a session with a personal trainer or research a book or program that has helped others. Don't feel like you have to set crazy expectations. Just *move*, 30 minutes a day.

#3: Eat Healthy. "Healthy" for me means at least 20 grams of protein and no more than 30 grams of carbs per meal, and 3 cups of vegetables a day (it's not as much as you think). Potatoes don't count. I'm talking greens, squash, carrots, peppers, tomatoes, broccoli, green beans, cauliflower. Cooked or raw, doesn't matter. Just get some color in your diet. How many meals a day do you need? It depends on your goals. Work with a nutritionist or doctor to figure out what's right for you. I usually do three meals a day, plus a snack like jicama or peppers with baba ganoush, berries and low-fat cottage cheese, or broccoli broiled with a little cheese and salt-free everything bagel seasoning!

#4: Meditate. Not everyone can sit crossed-legged in silence for hours on end. If you can, great! If not, start with just 5 minutes. Work up to 10, then 15, then 20. Think of it like the one part of a day where you don't have to answer to anyone - not even yourself. Just give yourself permission to not think, not plot, not process. Practice *being*, then staying, in the moment, without thinking about the past or the future. If you can't stand the sound of silence, check out guided meditations on YouTube, or use an app like Journey or Headspace.

#5: Hydrate. If I have a headache or feel off, I'm usually dehydrated. I start with the bare minimum: two pint glasses of water a day, which is 32 ounces. I have one when I wake up, and one at lunch. It's not that hard to do, and it's actually way less water than what I *should* be drinking. Ideally I'm getting a lot more throughout the day (*technically* I should be getting something in the 70-ounce+ zone), but sometimes I just forget or don't get around to it. Coffee, juice/wine and soda don't count!

#6: Take Your Vitamins. We can't always get the nutrients we need from the foods we eat, and some of us need to supplement. Talk to a doctor or nutritionist about your vitamin and mineral needs to make sure your levels support your lifestyle. I take fish oil, Vitamin D, Calcium, and an Emergency-C packet if I get a sore throat or tickle in my ear. Sometimes it nips a cold in the bud!

#7: Be Grateful. Don't laugh - this is a Great 8 for a reason! When I'm feeling slighted or disappointed or resentful about something, it's usually because my ego is in control and on a rampage. A quick way to keep it in check is to stop, take a minute, and focus on what I am thankful for. I embrace the moment I'm in - this moment, right now, and what I have, or am experiencing or can enjoy, that I couldn't have, experience, or enjoy a month ago, a year ago, a decade ago. Feeling gratitude in the present moment is one of the most powerful things you can do not just for yourself, but for the world around you. A grateful person isn't cruel or selfish. Today, find a moment, and use it to make a short list of five things that you either have or can do, that not everyone can have or do, that make your life happier, healthier, or easier. Be thankful now, right now, for where you have been or where you can go, and hold that feeling of gratitude in the present moment.

#8: Practice Self-Care. Okay, I see where you're going, but sleeping, eating healthy, and hydrating don't *also* count for this one. Self-Care is not just getting enough rest and putting good food in your body. Self-Care for me means taking a moment to be kind to myself, to appreciate myself, to forgive myself, and to celebrate myself. To practice your own Self-Care, you don't have to buy anything; you don't have to embark on anything or achieve anything. You can just take a moment once a day to give yourself something you need, even if it's just permission, or a break outside in the sunshine, or a round of applause for a job well done. Yes, it's great that you are improving your health, but if underneath that desire to be healthy isn't an even stronger desire to take *care* of yourself, you're going to burn out. So give yourself the TLC you need. It's okay. In fact, it'll be really good for you.

These Great Eight are my go-tos when I'm starting to get a little wobbly. When I'm doing them all, every day, I'm better. My life is better.

And when I really want to shine, I have a number 9...

NUMBER 9 (HOW TO SHINE)

After months of getting better and better at dialing in my routine, I started to feel like my Great Eight were the exact tools I needed to keep myself on track. I was losing weight, getting fitter, my stress levels were dropping and my mind felt even clearer and calmer than I'd ever felt in my life.

Still, there was something missing. I was achieving all my personal goals, but kept feeling like I was forgetting something important.

I was within 5 pounds of my goal weight when I signed up to take Yale University's "The Science of Well-Being" class through Coursera. Wow. What a class! After taking it, I realized exactly what I needed to do to close the gap. I'd found my #9 - **Connect With Others.**

In the rush to personal independence, we can forget that human beings are social animals. We might not always like it, but people need people. Isolated thanks to COVID-19, I couldn't help but realize how important it is to connect daily with at least one other human - if only to remind myself that I'm not alone.

If you're not a social butterfly, or part of a big family, it may be hard to connect with others. You may live in a remote area, or always be moving from one city to another. But if you want your life to truly be rich, you have to find a way to connect with other human beings. It's one of the best things you can do - not just for your life, but for other people's lives as well.

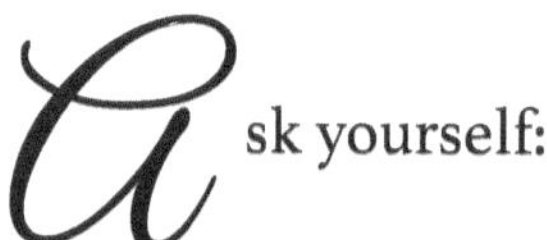sk yourself:

- *When was the last time you were kind to someone? (For clarity, **being kind** is the opposite of **being a dick**)*
- *When was the last time you shared a positive experience with another person? It doesn't have to be climbing a mountain with your bestie - it can be laughing in a checkout line with a stranger!*
- *When was the last time you thanked someone, or, better, yet, told them how thankful you were for them doing something, or for just being in your life?*
- *When was the last time you did something for someone else, not out of duty or obligation, but for the sheer pleasure of making someone's day better or life easier?*

All of these ways to Connect With Others are within your reach. Use today to take one step, with one other human.

ou can do this.

Seriously. You can. It's **possible.**

Thousands and thousands of people have done this. They may have using different tools or different methods - some good, some bad - but losing weight isn't rocket science. My whole life, I thought it was, but trust me, **it's not.** There isn't a body or a fitness level that is only available to a select group of humans who are genetically blessed or independently wealthy. Your brain and body are plastic and can be reformed, rewired, and rebuilt to be what you want them to be.

It may not be easy, but it can be simple.

Below are some of my favorite foods - my shortcuts and standards that made all this work a heck of a lot simpler. I always try to buy organic if I can afford it, and I always pick grass-fed beef or dairy products if they're available, because who needs hormones and chemicals adding an extra burden on top of what your body is already working hard to overcome?

Refer to Chapter 5 for my general approach to eating and Chapter 7 for my Food & Fitness Plan.

Note, the Chocolate and Vanilla meal replacement shakes I used ("Wio PRO-22, Phase 1-3") are typically only purchasable through a doctor, but here is the manufacturer website and nutritional profile, if you prefer to use an alternate meal replacement shake on your plan and want to match its nutritional profile: https://www.e-medtek.com/wio-mrp-meal-replacement-protocol-shake-vanilla-pro-22-phase-1-3-21-serving-bag

Always consult a doctor before starting a new diet or fitness plan. It not only ensures your health and safety; it gives you someone invested in your success that you can hold yourself accountable to!

Lastly, see the Appendix for recipes, indicated by italics and an asterisk *like this**

EASY HEALTHY PROTEIN CHOICES

- Eggs/Egg Whites - boiled, scrambled, or pan-fried with spray oil
- Pre-Roasted Whole Chicken from Whole Foods/Safeway/Sprouts
- Prepared Fresh or Frozen Salmon, Shrimp, Turkey, Grass-Fed Beef or Buffalo/Bison burgers
- Canned Wild-Caught Tuna or Salmon
- Chicken or Grass-Fed Pork or Beef sausages or hot dogs (in moderation; read your labels, watch your portion size, and stick to low-sugar varieties)
- *Turkey-Pork Meatballs or Mini Meatloaves**
- *Homemade Seafood Cakes**

EASY HEALTHY SNACK CHOICES

- Nancy's Probiotic Low-fat 2% Cottage Cheese with Strawberries, Raspberries, Blackberries or Blueberries
- Baba Ganoush (not Hummus), *Thai Peanut Sauce and Dip** or *Spicy Greek Yogurt Dip** with Jicama, Bell Peppers, Carrots, or Celery
- *Parmesan Everything Taco with Veggies**

- Small or Medium Apples with 1 Tablespoon of All-Natural Peanut or Almond Butter
- Plums or Apricots or Clementines with a Poached, Scrambled, or Hard-boiled Egg
- Freshé Canned Tuna Snacks (https://freshemeals.com)
- Whisps Cheese Crisps (watch your portion size)
- Lorissa's Kitchen Beef/Turkey/Chicken Jerkies (read your labels, watch your portion size and stick to low-sugar varieties)

EASY HEALTHY VEGGIE + CARB SWAPS

- Cascadian Farms Frozen Cauliflower Rice Blends
- Super Spinach by Organic Girl or any pre-washed Spinach/Baby Kale Blend
- "Zoodles" (zucchini noodles)
- Bell Peppers (all colors)
- Onions (all kinds)
- Mushrooms (all kinds)
- Zucchini, Yellow Squash, Broccoli or Cauliflower
- Green Beans, Shishito Peppers, or Asparagus
- Leafy and Cruciferous Greens - Kale, Spinach, Chard, Cabbage, Collards
- *Easy Roast Veggies**
- *Super Salad Mix**
- *Cauliflower Rice**
- *Baked Spaghetti Squash**
- *Roasted Sweet Potato or Zucchini Fries**
- *Stir-Fried Stalks**

EASY HEALTHY FATS + CONDIMENTS

- Olive Oil
- Avocado
- Grass-Fed Butter
- Cheeses or Nut Butters (Cheeses and Nut Butters are so calorie-dense, I find I have to treat them like a Fat)
- Primal Palate Salad Dressings
- Bolthouse Farms Yogurt Salad Dressings
- Flavored Oil/Vinegar combos, like those available at Amphora Nueva (https://amphoranueva.com)
- Frontier Green Harvest Seasoning Blend
- Savory Spice Shop Seasonings (https://www.savoryspiceshop.com/)
- Real Salt Garlic Salt

QUICK MEALS AND TREATS

- *Buffalo Chicken Casserole**
- *Faux Blueberry Danish**
- *Kitchen Sink Curry**
- *Stuffed Peppers with Cauliflower Rice Filling**
- *Spaghetti Squash Pizza**
- *Dat Keto Lady's PB Cheesecake Bars (via YouTube)*

** See Recipe Appendix*

RESOURCES FOR MORE RECIPES

Below are some of my favorite resources for low-carb recipes. **Note:** When using "Keto" recipes, keep in mind that while they are typically low in carbohydrates, they are often high in fat, so you need to be mindful of the *calories* you're consuming, not just the *carbs*. Losing weight, in my experience, requires reducing both calorie *and* carb consumption. Pay attention to both!

WEBSITES WITH LOW-CARB RECIPES:

- https://nomnompaleo.com
- https://www.wholesomeyum.com
- https://minimalistbaker.com/
- https://alldayidreamaboutfood.com/
- https://drdavinahseats.com
- https://www.sugarfreemom.com
- https://www.castironketo.net/
- https://www.wholekitchensink.com
- https://allthehealthythings.com

COOKBOOKS TO INSPIRE YOU

- Milk Street Fast and Slow
- Cook This Not That
- The Frugal Paleo Cookbook
- Naturally Sweet
- Skinny Taste One & Done
- Dinner In An Instant
- Korean Paleo

APPENDIX: MY GO-TO RECIPES

PROTEIN

Turkey-Pork Meatballs or Mini Meatloaves

This is the mix I use when I make "Cheeseburger Salad" - my go-to satisfier when I'm craving In-N-Out. I make 4-oz hamburger patties and broil a slice of Cheddar cheese on top, then slice the burger up and toss it with my Super Salad mix, halved cherry tomatoes, and Primal Palate Thousand Island Dressing.

1/2 lb ground turkey (thigh meat is best)

1/2 lb ground pork

2 cloves minced garlic

1 Tbsp Onion Chutney (optional)

1 Tbsp minced red onion

1 tsp Worcestershire sauce

1/2 tsp each salt and pepper

1 large egg

1/4 cup Panko-style Italian Seasoned breadcrumbs

In a bowl with your hands or a mixer (dough hook attachment; low speed), combine all ingredients. Using an ice cream or cookie scoop, form into large or small balls. Bake in regular muffin tins for mini meatloaves (375 degrees for 15-20 mins) or mini-muffin tins for meatballs (375 degrees for 10-15 minutes). Alternatively, shape into patties and pan-fry. Always cook to an internal temperature of 165 degrees.

Homemade Seafood Cakes

I adapted this from Michelle Tam's Spicy Tuna Cakes (https:// nomnompaleo.com/post/91332244628/spicy-tuna-cakes), which are also delicious!

2 tablespoons coconut oil, melted

10 oz. canned water-packed tuna, salmon, or crab, drained

2 Tbsp finely chopped green onion

2 Tbsp finely chopped red onion

2 Tbsp finely chopped parsley

1 cup mashed baked sweet potato

finely grated zest from ½ medium lemon

1 tablespoon minced red pepper

2 large eggs

½ teaspoon red chili sauce or Sriracha

1 tsp salt

Freshly ground black pepper to taste

Mix everything together by hand (this is important because you don't want the fish or crab chunks to be too broken up). Press 1/4 cup portions into a non-stick muffin tin and bake at 350 degrees for 20 minutes OR form into patties and cook in batches in a non-stick pan with a little bit of coconut oil, ghee, or olive oil.

Thai Peanut Sauce and Dip

This sauce has a lot of ingredients but I use it for everything - on grilled chicken, as a dressing for Asian coleslaw, to dip spring rolls in, or even just on spaghetti squash or zoodles with pan-fried tofu cubes or shrimp.

1/4 cup lime juice

3 Tbsp unseasoned rice vinegar

1/4 cup peanut or avocado oil

1/2 cup creamy unsweetened peanut butter

2-3 Tbsp soy sauce (depending on how salty you like it)

1/4 cup "golden" monkfruit sweetener, like Lakanto

2 Tbsp fresh minced ginger

1 Tbsp powdered ginger

1 1/2 Tbsp fresh minced garlic

2 tsp Red Boat Fish Sauce

2 Tbsp toasted sesame oil

1/2 tsp sriracha

Mix all ingredients with a whisk or by pulsing in a blender. For Asian coleslaw, mix dressing 1/2 cup at a time with one bag of broccoli slaw plus an extra cup each of shredded red cabbage, shredded carrots, and julienne sliced red, orange, or yellow bell peppers. A little sauce goes a long way!

Spicy Greek Yogurt Dip aka "Fry Sauce"

I love Savory Spice Shop's "Dip, Dip, Hooray" set, which has a bunch of seasonings you can just mix into nonfat or low-fat Greek yogurt. This dip is a little more work but I love it with Roasted Sweet

Potato or Zucchini Fries, cooked shrimp, or, if you mix in a little dill relish and minced onion, Homemade Seafood Cakes.

1/2 cup ketchup

1/2 cup tomato sauce

1 Tbsp tomato paste

1 tsp powdered erythritol or granulated monkfruit sweetener

2 tsp lemon juice

2 tsp red chili sauce or sriracha

2 tsp prepared horseradish

2 tsp Worcestershire sauce

1/4 cup mayonnaise

1 cup nonfat Greek yogurt

Stir all ingredients together until well-combined. Keep refrigerated.

Low-Salt Everything Bagel Seasoning

2 Tbsp each white and black sesame seeds

1 Tbsp dried minced onion

1 Tbsp dried minced garlic (I like Jane's Crazy Chunky Garlic Seasoning or Lesley Elizabeth's Oh So Garlic Seasoning)

2 tsp poppy seeds

Mix above together and store at room temperature in a sealed container or shaker.

Parmesan Everything Taco with Veggies

*If you don't have a taco shell mold, you can make these in giant muffin tins or just drape the cooked cheese over a half a bell pepper or a bowl of steamed broccoli (or, if you're feeling ambitious, half a bell pepper **stuffed** with steamed broccoli!).*

2 Tbsp to 1/4 cup grated Parmesan cheese

1/2 tsp low-salt (above) or no-salt (store bought) Everything Bagel Seasoning

Diced or shredded bell peppers, carrots, jicama, avocado, or shredded red cabbage

Heat a small frying pan on medium heat, and sprinkle the Parmesan evenly over it. Let the Parmesan melt a little, then sprinkle the Everything Bagel Seasoning over it evenly. When the bottom of the Parmesan is evenly browned, use a spatula to lift it up and slide it on top of a taco mold or thin glass bottle to cool. Fill with fresh veggies.

VEGGIES

Easy Roast Veggies

I rely a lot on bell peppers, zucchini, summer squash, and onions when I am trying to fill my plate with vegetables - I slice and sauté them together, or chop and roast them. This recipe is adapted from Ina Garten's "Vegetable Tian" recipe. If you like the taste, try adding 1/2 cup chopped fennel to the onion/garlic mixture!

1 Tbsp olive oil

1 cup diced red or yellow onion

1 tsp minced fresh garlic

1 medium or 2 small zucchini

1 medium or 2 small yellow squash

3-4 roma tomatoes

1/2 cup Parmesan or Gruyere cheese, grated

2 tsp Italian seasoning or fresh thyme

Salt + black pepper, to taste

Slice all the vegetables into thin coins, like thick poker chips. Sauté the onion and garlic (and 1/2 cup diced fennel, if desired)

in the olive oil. When tender and translucent, remove from heat and spread the mixture in the bottom of a casserole pan. Preheat oven to 400 degrees. Take the sliced veggies and line them up in the pan on top of the onion mixture like rows of Oreos, alternating them like you would for a barbecue veggie kabob - tomato, zucchini, squash, tomato, zucchini, squash, etc. If you want to be extra fancy you can arrange in a spiral! Sprinkle the casserole with salt and pepper and Italian seasoning or fresh thyme. Cover with foil and bake 20 minutes. Remove foil, add cheese on top of vegetables, then bake another 10-15 minutes, until cheese is lightly browned.

Super Salad Mix

I eat this just about every other week. It's colorful and easy and I can use it as a base for most dressing/protein combinations.

1-2 small clamshells pre-washed "Super Spinach" or Spinach/Baby Kale Blend (*alternatively, you can wash and tear up 6 cups of red leaf lettuce, but don't use Spring Mix because it tends to go bad quickly*)

1/2 a head of a red cabbage, shredded (about 2 cups)

2 cups shredded carrots

Mix above in a giant Ziploc bag and keep in fridge. Makes 3 servings.

Super Salad Combinations: *Store-bought Roasted Chicken and Low-Sugar Italian or Balsamic Dressing; Pork/Turkey Meatballs or burgers with Broiled Sharp Cheddar Slice + Chopped Tomatoes + Primal Palate Thousand Island Dressing; Grilled Steak + Pico de Gallo + Avocado + Chipotle Ranch or Caesar Dressing mixed with 1/4 tsp Taco seasoning; Grilled Chicken Bratwurst or Polish Sausage + Sauerkraut + sautéed Bell Peppers + Primal Palate Honey Mustard Dressing*

Cauliflower Rice

I generally buy pre-made fresh or frozen cauliflower rice because it's worth the convenience to me, but if you want to make it yourself, you can use a box grater or the shredding attachment on your food processor. I use cauliflower rice not as a substitute for white rice by itself (I grew up Asian so there really is no substitute for me, to be honest!) but it is great as a filler, thickener, or base ingredient for just about any soup or casserole.

If you're craving something comforting, add a pat of butter, a tablespoon of Greek yogurt or Heavy Cream, a tablespoon of Parmesan or Pecorino/Romano, some garlic salt and lemon pepper to a cup or two of hot Cauliflower Rice. It's not that high in calories and mimics the texture of risotto (you can do the same with Baked Spaghetti Squash). Denise Bustard also has some great ideas for flavored versions of Cauliflower Rice on her website: https:// sweetpeasandsaffron.com/cauliflower-rice-recipes/

Baked Spaghetti Squash

Spaghetti Squash is not something you can buy pre-made generally, and it's much better made fresh anyway. Look for a Spaghetti Squash that's about the size of a small Nerf football - 6-8 inches long. Slice it in half and scoop out the seeds inside. Prick all over the inside and outside with a fork and place cut side down on an aluminum foil- or parchment-lined baking sheet. Bake in a preheated 350 degree oven for 50-70 minutes. It's ready when the inside is slightly translucent but not mushy. Take the baked squash out of the oven, turn the halves cut side up on the pan, and let it cool 10 minutes, then use a fork to shred the insides into a bowl. Substitute for pasta or noodles in any recipe (e.g., Spaghetti Carbonara, Pad Thai, Cincinnati Chili, Linguine with Clams, etc.). You can even skip the shredding step and just fill the baked spaghetti squash with your favorite pasta sauce. Dr. G. swears by Trader Joe's Almond Turmeric Dressing!

Roasted Sweet Potato or Zucchini Fries

It's no secret that oven-roasted veggie fries - while not the same thing as their deep-fried doppelgängers - are still pretty satisfying. One of my favorite carb indulgences is Panko-style breadcrumbs. They are pretty high in carbs (20g or so for 1/4 cup) so they are definitely a treat, but if it's a gym day or I am pairing them with enough fat, fiber, and protein, I know I can indulge without worrying I'm spiking my blood sugar. Note: if you are trying to restrict your carbs, you can try "keto" or "paleo" substitutes for traditional Panko in this recipe.

3-4 Japanese Sweet Potatoes or Zucchini, cut into french-fry-sized pieces (about 3 cups' worth)

4 Tbsp olive oil

3 Tbsp Panko-style Italian seasoned breadcrumbs

2 Tbsp grated Parmesan cheese

1/2 tsp garlic salt

1/2 tsp garlic powder

1/2 tsp fresh ground pepper *or* lemon pepper

1/2 tsp dried parsley

1 tsp Frontier Spice Company's "Green Harvest" seasoning

Preheat your oven to 450 degrees. Toss the cut-up vegetables with the olive oil in a large bowl until evenly coated. In a separate bowl, mix the remaining ingredients together, then toss this mixture with the oil-coated veggies. Spread the veggies out on a cooling rack positioned on top of an aluminum foil- or parchment-lined baking sheet (this is to allow air to circulate underneath the "fries" and avoid them sticking to and burning on the baking sheet). Bake 25-30 minutes until breadcrumbs are golden brown. Drizzle with Spicy Greek Yogurt Dip like nachos!

Stir-Fried Stalks

This recipe is adapted from one that Dr. G. swears is perfect for munching on instead of salty buttered popcorn!

1 to 1 1/2 Tbsp soy sauce (to taste)

1 tsp sesame oil

1/2 to 1 tsp fresh grated garlic (to taste)

1/2 to 1 tsp fresh grated ginger (to taste)

1/4 tsp Red Boat Fish Sauce

1/2 tsp rice vinegar or lemon juice

20-30 green beans or 1 bunch asparagus (about as much as you can hold in two hands)

Whisk together first 5 ingredients in a small bowl. Add green beans or asparagus to a wide saucepan, plus 1 Tbsp water. Cover with a lid and steam stalks briefly in the pan until they just turn bright green but are still crisp. Remove lid, pour soy mixture over stalks and sauté 2-3 more minutes until tender.

MEALS

Buffalo Chicken Casserole Dip

I was almost 30 lbs down when the holidays hit, and didn't want to derail, so I brought this to potlucks to have something high-protein and low-carb to snack on instead of 7-Layer Dip with Tortilla Chips. It's great with celery sticks or bell pepper "scoops" and I often eat it as a meal because it's so filling!

2 cups pre-roasted cauliflower*

3 Tbsp butter

4 cloves garlic, minced

1/2 cup diced red onion

1/2 cup diced carrot

1 cup diced celery

1/2 cup chicken broth

1 8-oz block Neufchâtel cream cheese, at room temperature

1/4 cup nonfat plain Greek yogurt

1 tsp dried mustard powder

2 Tbsp chopped fresh parsley

1/2 cup diced red bell pepper

3/4 cup Frank's Red Hot Sauce

2 cups diced pre-cooked rotisserie chicken

2 cups shredded cheddar cheese

1/2 cup blue cheese crumbles

1/2 cup sliced green onions

In a large saucepan, melt butter, then add onion, garlic, carrot, and celery. Cook until soft. Add chicken broth, give it a stir, then remove from heat and stir in cream cheese until melted and all blended together. Sir in Greek yogurt, mustard powder, parsley, diced peppers, then Frank's Red Hot Sauce. Fold in cauliflower, chicken, and 1 cup of the cheddar cheese. Spread mixture into a casserole and top with remaining cheddar. Bake for 15 minutes in a 350 degree oven, till top is brown and bubbling. Top with blue cheese crumbles and bake 5 more minutes. Remove from oven and top with blue cheese and green onions.

To roast cauliflower, preheat oven to 450 degrees. Cut up a whole cauliflower into malt-ball size pieces and arrange on a sheet pan. Spray with cooking spray (I use my "Misto" olive oil sprayer) and sprinkle with salt and pepper. Roast for 15-20 minutes, depending on how browned you like it. Makes approximately 4 cups.

Kitchen Sink Curry

*Many Indian, Thai, and Vietnamese curries contain cauliflower or squash, and are served over a bed of rice. Even basmati rice is pretty high in carbs, so I found myself making the same curries without these veggies, then serving them **on top of** steamed or roasted cauliflower or squash **instead** of rice. It gave me the same flavors with less carbs!*

1-2 lbs raw turkey or chicken, chopped into 1-inch cubes

1 tsp sea salt

3 tsp Madras, Red, Green, or Yellow Curry Powder or Paste*

2 Tbsp olive or coconut oil

2 minced garlic cloves

1 cup chopped onion

3/4 cup to 1 cup liquid (water, broth, or coconut milk)

2 cups fresh vegetables, cut into 1/2—inch chunks (Roma tomatoes, carrots, peeled sweet potatoes, pumpkin, bell peppers, broccoli, green peas, spinach)

Rub chicken pieces all over with curry powder and salt, making sure to coat well. Heat a skillet over medium-high heat and add the oil. When it's hot, brown the chicken cubes on all sides, then add the garlic, onion, and liquid. Bring to a boil, then reduce the heat to a simmer and add remaining vegetables. Cover and braise for about 25 minutes until the chicken is cooked through (add more liquid halfway through if needed). Serve on a bed of roasted or steamed cauliflower or squash (I like acorn, butternut, zucchini, or summer squash).

**Check out Savory Spice Shop's "Curry Up" or "Thai Fecta" Spice*

Sets, or Oaktown Spice Shop's Persian Lime Curry Rub, or Jamaican or Japanese Curry Powders for a nice change from traditional curries.

Stuffed Peppers with Cauliflower Rice Filling

I make these with cauliflower rice instead of regular rice, and vary the protein (try diced grass-fed hot dogs, shredded chicken, or Italian sausage), the seasonings (you can substitute taco or Italian seasoning for the chili seasoning) and the cheese to suit whatever flavors you're in the mood for. It's an easy-to-make, healthy hot lunch or dinner that reheats beautifully the next day. You can even try these Philly Cheese Stuffed Bell Peppers if you're feeling ambitious: https://www. castironketo.net/blog/keto-philly-cheese-steak-stuffed-peppers/

3 cups fresh or defrosted cauliflower rice

1 Tbsp olive oil

3 cloves garlic, minced

1/2 cup diced red or yellow onion

1/2 cup diced green onion

1 cup diced zucchini (optional)

4 large bell peppers, cut in half with seeds removed

1 lb ground lean beef or bison

1 Tbsp chili seasoning

2 Tbsp ketchup

2 cups shredded Cheddar or Mexican Blend cheese

Preheat oven to 375 degrees. Line the peppers in a casserole pan side by side, cut side up. In a large saucepan, heat oil, garlic, onions, zucchini (if using) and chili seasoning until onion is soft. Add beef and ketchup, and sauté until meat is cooked through, stirring frequently. Add salt and pepper to taste, then add cauliflower rice and stir. Put the lid on the saucepan to "steam" the cauliflower rice for 1 minute (if using defrosted cauliflower rice, skip this step). Once cauliflower is heated through, taste and adjust seasonings, adding salt and pepper as needed. Stuff peppers with mixture and top with shredded cheese. Bake 30 minutes, then broil for 5-10 minutes to brown cheese. Serve with red/green onion, avocado, fresh cilantro, pico de gallo, and Greek yogurt instead of sour cream.

Spaghetti Squash Pizza

This is maybe my favorite "diet" hack - it's high in protein, way lower in carbs than regular pizza, and satisfies my craving when I just need some gooey cheese and crispy pepperoni for dinner.

3 cups pre-cooked Spaghetti Squash

1 1/2 cups Low-fat Cottage Cheese (optional)

1 Tbsp Pizza Seasoning or Italian Seasoning

1 1/2 cups Pizza or Spaghetti Sauce

2 cups shredded Italian or Pizza Cheese Blend

1 1/2 cups Pizza Toppings (Pepperoni, thin-sliced Mushrooms, Bell Peppers, Black Olives, Sun-Dried Tomatoes and Basil, Barbecued Chicken and Green Onions, Bacon and Pineapple)

2 Tbsp Parmesan cheese, grated

Preheat oven to 350 degrees. Lightly coat the bottom of a casserole pan with olive oil and spread Spaghetti Squash in pan in a single layer. Top with cottage cheese, then sprinkle Pizza/Italian Seasoning on top. Spread Pizza or Spaghetti sauce over the cottage cheese layer, then top with shredded cheese blend. Finish with the toppings you want, sprinkle with the Parmesan, and bake for 20-30 minutes, until cheese is bubbly.

Faux Blueberry Danish

I made this at home after going to a farmer's market and staring longingly at the fresh blueberry cheese danishes in a bakery stall. I knew if I had even one of those danishes, it would become a weekly habit, so I came up with this recipe to derail my craving!

1 package Paleo/Keto Blueberry Muffin Mix (such as Lakanto or Miss Jones Baking Co.), plus preparation ingredients (will vary depending on mix)

3/4 cup fresh blueberries

8 ounces cream cheese, softened

3 Tbsp powdered sugar substitute (like Swerve or Lakanto monkfruit)

1 large egg

1/2 tsp vanilla extract

Mix cream cheese, sugar substitute, egg and vanilla; set aside. Prepare muffin mix as directed on package and stir in 1/2 cup of fresh blueberries. Fill muffin cups or muffin top pan with batter; top with two tablespoons of cream cheese mixture and remaining blueberries. Bake as directed on package.

Fresh Fruit Coffee Cake

Despite being truly happier with my "new normal," some-times I do want to feel like the "old" me - the one who used to bring a coffee cake to brunch and have a slice with a friend without feeling guilty. When I'm nostalgic, I make this lower-sugar version, which is tasty enough for everyone to enjoy with a cup of tea or cappuccino.

3/4 cup blanched fine almond flour

3/4 cup Arrowhead Mills Protein Flour

1 tsp cinnamon

1/4 tsp mace (can substitute nutmeg)

1/4 tsp ginger

1/8 tsp ground cardamom

8 Tbsp softened unsalted butter

1 cup Whole Earth Allulose Baking Blend

1 egg

1 tsp vanilla or vanilla bean paste

1/2 cup half-and-half

(optional) 1 Tbsp "golden" monkfruit blend

1 pound fresh stone fruit or baking apples (plums, pluots, apricots, peaches, nectarines)

Preheat oven to 350 degrees and grease a 9" springform pan. In one bowl, whisk together the flours and spices. In a separate (bigger) bowl, beat the butter and allulose blend together till fluffy. Add the egg and vanilla and blend well, then add half the flour mixture, then 1/4 cup of the half-and-half, then the rest of the flour mixture, then the rest of the half-and-half. Spread in the pan, then top with the fresh fruit and, if you like, a sprinkle of golden monkfruit blend on top. Bake for 45-55 minutes, until golden brown on top and set in the center. Let cool 5 minutes, then run a knife around the edge to loosen the cake from the springform pan. Remove the outer ring, then late cake finish cooling completely.

ABOUT THE AUTHOR

Diagnosed with Stage 3 triple negative breast cancer at 34, doctors told her she had a 1 in 3 chance of making it to 40 without a recurrence. Intent on making the next 6 years count, Capil embarked on a "40-by-40" bucket list, which included running the NYC Marathon, skydiving in Colorado, kayaking the Main Salmon River, rock-climbing in Moab, seeing an Oprah Winfrey show, going on a chocolate tour of Paris, swimming with dolphins, learning how to figure skate, and climbing Mt. Kilimanjaro, among other things. Capil not only checked off everything on her list; she is still cancer-free eleven years later, and hard at work on a "50-by-50."

In addition to a memoir of walking the Camino Santiago in 2018 (*Camino de Lemon*) and the first in a YA fiction trilogy (*The Underground*), Capil is the author of three books on crisis management (*Recipe for Lemonade*), disaster recovery (*Life After Lemonade*, also available as an Audible.com audiobook), and post-traumatic growth (*New Tricks*).

Read more about author April Capil at www.aprilcapil.com or check out her other e-books on Smashwords.com.

You can also purchase print copies of any of the above books (including this one) at most online retailers.